Vegetables & Sides Dash Diet Slow Cooker Recipes

Healthy & Fit Every Day

with These Recipes

Carmela Rojas

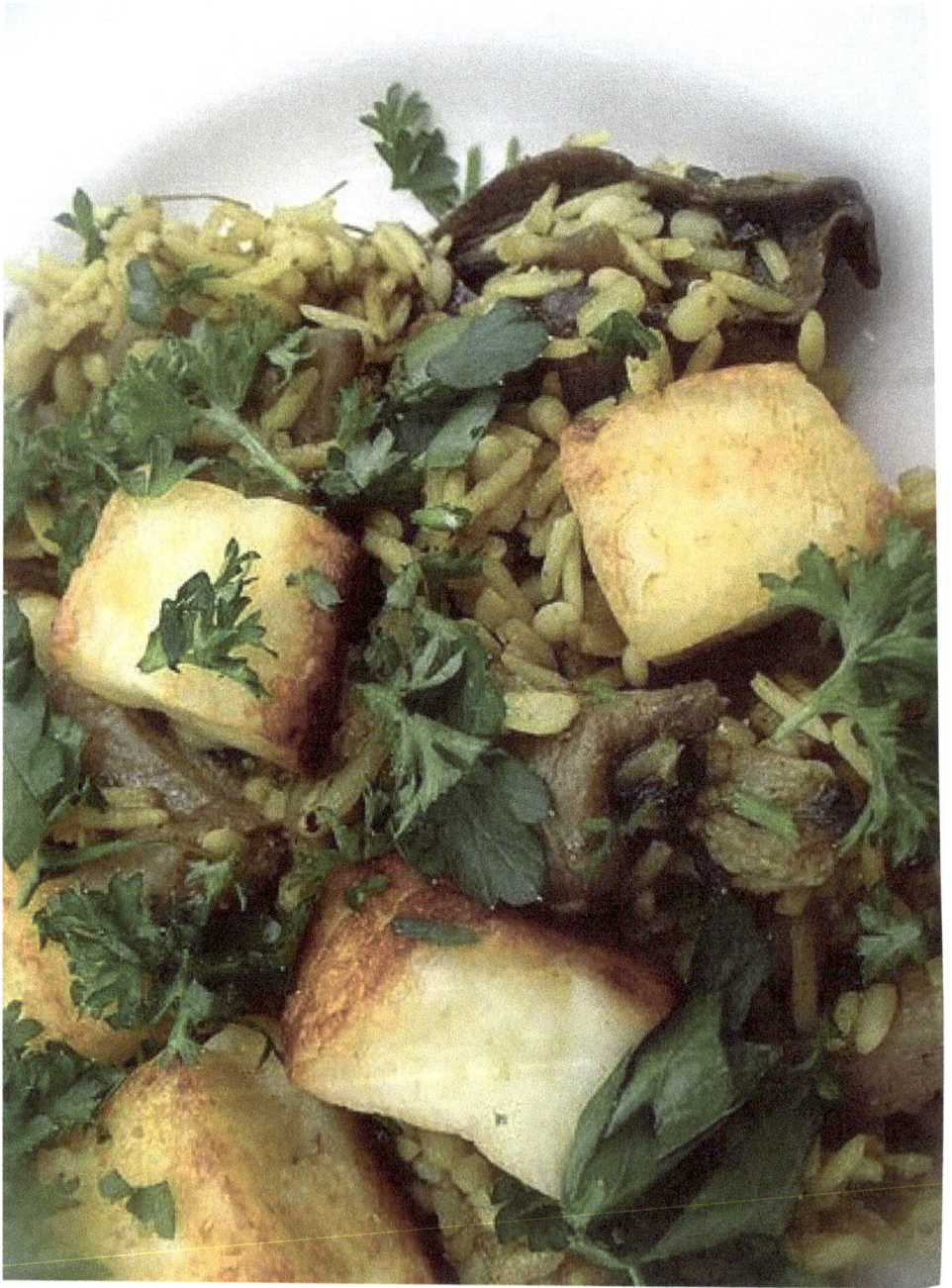

TABLE OF CONTENTS

Pilaf with Bella Mushrooms

Servings: 6

Cooking Time: 3 Hours

Ingredients:

- 1 cup wild rice
- 6 green onions, chopped
- ½ pound baby Bella mushrooms
- 2 cups water
- 2 tablespoons olive oil
- 2 garlic cloves, minced

Directions:

1. In your slow cooker, mix the rice with garlic, onions, oil, mushrooms and water, toss, cover and cook on Low for 3 hours.
2. Stir the pilaf one more time, divide between plates and serve.

Nutrition Info:

Calories 151, Fat 5.1g, Cholesterol 0mg, Sodium 9mg, Carbohydrate 23.3g, Fiber 2.6g, Sugars 1.7g, Protein 5.2g, Potassium 343mg

Italian Style Yellow Squash

Servings: 6

Cooking Time: 6 Hours

Ingredients:

- 2 cups zucchinis, sliced
- 1 teaspoon Italian seasoning
- 1 teaspoon garlic powder
- 2 tablespoons olive oil
- 2 cups yellow squash, peeled and cut into wedges
- Black pepper to the taste

Directions:

1. Grease the slow cooker with the oil, add zucchini, squash, Italian seasoning, black pepper and garlic powder, toss well, cover, cook on Low for 6 hours, divide between plates and serve as a side dish.

Nutrition Info:

Calories 61, Fat 5.2g, Cholesterol 1mg, Sodium 51mg, Carbohydrate 3.7g, Fiber 1.1g, Sugars 1.7g, Protein 1g, Potassium 104mg

Slow Cooker Chili Rellenos

Servings: 4 Servings

Ingredients:

- 4 ounces (115 g) whole green chilies
- 1 cup (115 g) grated Cheddar cheese
- 1 cup (115 g) grated Monterey Jack cheese
- 1 large tomato, sliced
- 4 eggs, separated
- ¾ cup (175 ml) evaporated milk
- 2 tablespoons (16 g) flour

Directions:

1. Spray sides and bottom of slow cooker with nonstick cooking spray. Remove seeds from chilies; cut into strips. Place half of chilies on bottom of slow cooker. Layer with Cheddar cheese, rest of chilies, Monterey Jack cheese, and tomato slices. Beat egg whites until stiff. Fold in slightly beaten yolks, milk, and flour. Pour over top of tomatoes in the pot. Cover and cook on high for 2 to 3 hours.

Nutrition Info:

Per serving: 165 g water; 427 calories (63% from fat, 26% from protein, 11% from carb); 28 g protein; 30 g total fat; 17 g saturated fat; 9 g monounsaturated fat; 2 g polyunsaturated fat; 12 g carb; 1 g fiber; 2 g sugar; 536 mg phosphorus; 642 mg calcium; 2 mg iron; 545 mg sodium; 417 mg potassium; 1481 IU vitamin A; 226 mg ATE vitamin E; 30 mg vitamin C; 315 mg cholesterol

Stevia Peas with Marjoram

Servings: 12

Cooking Time: 5 Hours

Ingredients:

- 1 pound carrots, sliced
- 1 yellow onion, chopped
- 16 ounces peas
- 2 tablespoons stevia
- 2 tablespoons olive oil
- 4 garlic cloves, minced
- ¼ cup water
- 1 teaspoon marjoram, dried
- A pinch of white pepper

Directions:

1. In your slow cooker, mix the carrots with water, onion, oil, stevia, garlic, marjoram, white pepper and peas, toss, cover and cook on High for 5 hours.
2. Divide between plates and serve as a side dish.

Nutrition Info:

Calories 71, Fat 2.5g, Cholesterol 0mg, Sodium 29mg, Carbohydrate 12.1g, Fiber 3.1g, Sugars 4.4g, Protein 2.5g, Potassium 231mg

Okra Mix

Servings: 4

Cooking Time: 3 Hours

Ingredients:

- 1 cup cherry tomatoes, halved
- 1 and ½ cups red onion, cut into wedges
- 2 cups okra, sliced
- 2 cups yellow bell pepper, chopped
- 1 cup mushrooms, sliced
- 2 and ½ cups zucchini, sliced
- 1 tablespoon thyme, chopped
- 2 tablespoons basil, chopped
- ½ cup olive oil
- ½ cup balsamic vinegar

Directions:

1. In a large bowl, mix onion with tomatoes, okra, zucchini, bell pepper, mushrooms, basil, thyme, oil and vinegar, cover and cook on High for 3 hours.
2. Divide between plates and serve as a side dish.

Nutrition Info:

Calories 304, Fat 25.8g, Cholesterol 0mg, Sodium 19mg, Carbohydrate 17.7g, Fiber 5.1g, Sugars 8.4g, Protein 3.9g, Potassium 703mg

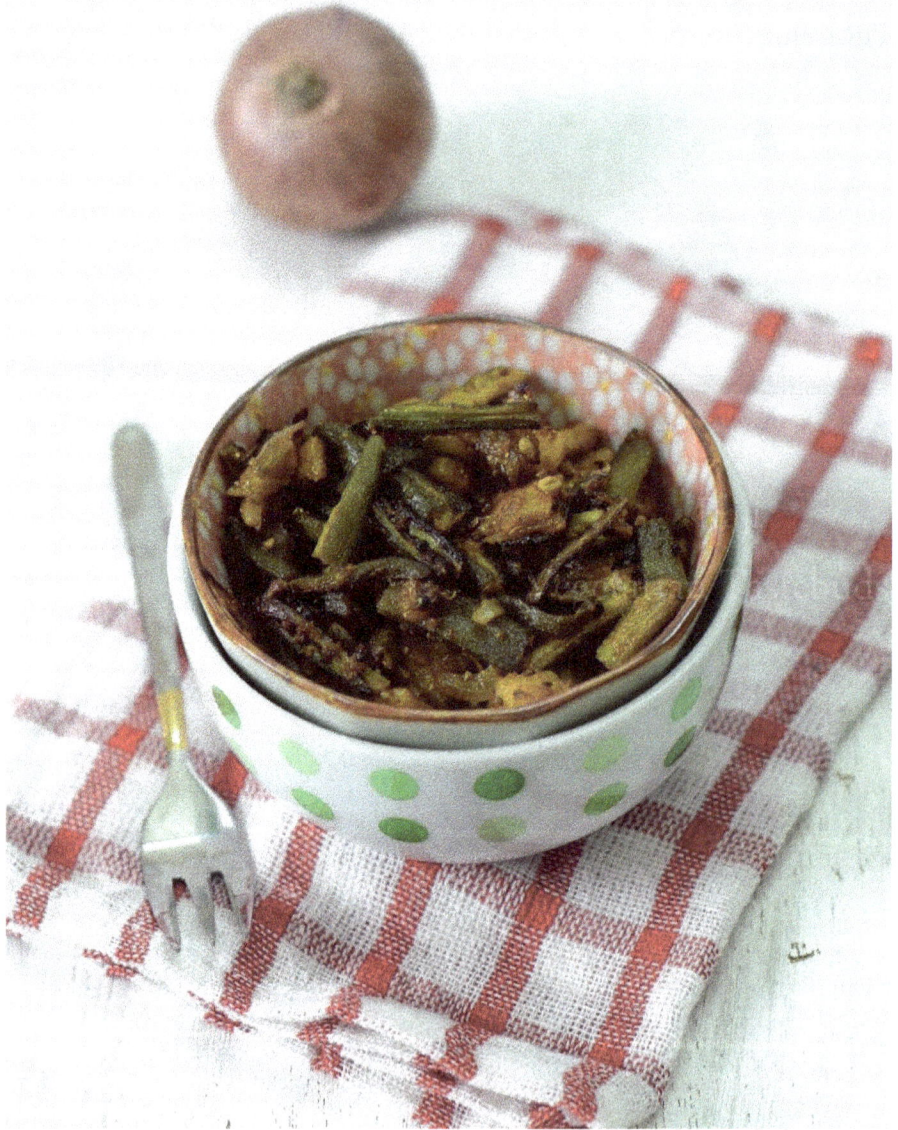

Parlsey Fennel

Servings: 4

Cooking Time: 2 Hours And 30 Minutes

Ingredients:

- 2 fennel bulbs, sliced
- Juice and zest of 1 lime
- 2 teaspoons avocado oil
- ½ teaspoon turmeric powder
- 1 tablespoon parsley, chopped
- ¼ cup veggie stock, low-sodium

Directions:

1. In slow cooker, combine the fennel with the lime juice, zest and the other ingredients, put the lid on and cook on Low for 2 hours and 30 minutes.
2. Divide between plates and serve as a side dish.

Nutrition Info:

Calories 47, Fat 0.6g, Cholesterol 0mg, Sodium 71mg, Carbohydrate 10.8g, Fiber 4.3g, Sugars 0.4g, Protein 1.7g, Potassium 521mg

Succotash

Servings: 12 Servings

Ingredients:

- 1 can (28 ounces, or 785 g) no-salt-added diced tomatoes, undrained
- 1 pound (455 g) frozen lima beans
- 1 pound (455 g) frozen corn
- 3 medium red potatoes, coarsely chopped
- ½ cup (120 ml) low-sodium chicken broth
- 1 teaspoon crushed thyme
- ¼ teaspoon black pepper

Directions:

1. In a 4- to 5-quart (3.8 to 4.8 L) slow cooker, combine undrained tomatoes, lima beans, corn, and potatoes. Add broth, thyme, and pepper. Cover and cook on low for 7 to 9 hours or on high for 3½ to 4½ hours.

Nutrition Info:

Per serving: 135 g water; 111 calories (3% from fat, 16% from protein, 81% from carb); 5 g protein; 0 g total fat; 0 g saturated fat; 0 g monounsaturated fat; 0 g polyunsaturated fat; 24 g carb;

5 g fiber; 3 g sugar; 92 mg phosphorus; 40 mg calcium; 3 mg iron; 30 mg sodium; 423 mg potassium; 146 IU vitamin A; 0 mg ATE vitamin E; 12 mg vitamin C; 0 mg cholesterol

Broccoli Rice Casserole

Servings: 4 Servings

Ingredients:

- 1 pound (455 g) frozen broccoli, cooked and drained
- 10 ounces (280 g) low-sodium cream of mushroom soup
- 1/3 cup (53 g) chopped onion
- 10 ounces (280 g) Swiss cheese, shredded
- ½ cup (120 ml) skim milk
- 1½ cups (248 g) cooked rice

Directions:

1. Mix everything together, leaving enough cheese to sprinkle over the top. Place in slow cooker and top with reserved cheese. Cook on low for 2 hours.

Nutrition Info:

Per serving: 270 g water; 437 calories (43% from fat, 25% from protein, 32% from carb); 27 g protein; 21 g total fat; 13 g saturated fat; 6 g monounsaturated fat; 1 g polyunsaturated fat; 35 g carb; 4 g fiber; 5 g sugar; 604 mg phosphorus; 797 mg calcium; 1 mg

iron; 338 mg sodium; 798 mg potassium; 1355 IU vitamin A; 170 mg ATE vitamin E; 102 mg vitamin C; 68 mg cholesterol

Italians Style Mushroom Mix

Servings: 6

Cooking Time: 4 Hours

Ingredients:

- 1 pound mushrooms, halved
- 1 teaspoon Italian seasoning
- 3 tablespoons olive oil
- 1 cup tomato sauce, no-salt-added
- 1 yellow onion, chopped

Directions:

1. In your slow cooker, mix the mushrooms with the oil, onion, Italian seasoning and tomato sauce, toss, cover and cook on Low for 4 hours.
2. Divide between plates and serve as a side dish.

Nutrition Info:

Calories96, Fat 7.5g, Cholesterol 1mg, Sodium 219mg, Carbohydrate 6.5g, Fiber 1.8g, Sugars 3.9g, Protein 3.1g, Potassium 403mg

Shallot And Mushrooms Mix

Servings: 8

Cooking Time: 8 Hours

Ingredients:

- 1 and ½ pounds cremini mushrooms, halved
- ½ cup coconut cream
- 2 garlic cloves, minced
- 1 shallot, chopped
- ¼ cup low sodium chicken stock
- 2 tablespoons parsley, chopped
- 1 teaspoon cornstarch

Directions:

1. In your slow cooker, mix the mushrooms with garlic, shallot, stock and parsley, cover and cook on Low for 7 hours.
2. Add coconut cream mixed with the cornstarch, cover, cook on Low for 1 more hour, divide between plates and serve as a side dish.

Nutrition Info:

Calories 62, Fat 3.7g, Cholesterol 0mg, Sodium 10mg, Carbohydrate 5.2g, Fiber 0.9g, Sugars 2g, Protein 2.6g, Potassium 433mg

Chili Beans

Servings: About 5

Cooking Time: 4 Hrs

Ingredients:

- 1 ½ cup chopped Bell Pepper
- 1 ½ cup sliced Mushrooms (white)
- 1 cup chopped Onion
- 1 tbsp. Olive Oil
- 1 tbsp. Chili Powder
- 2 chopped cloves Garlic
- 1 tsp. chopped Chipotle Chili
- ½ tsp. Cumin
- 15.5 oz drained Black Beans
- 1 cup diced Tomatoes (no salt)
- 2 tbsp. chopped Cilantro

Directions:

1. Place all the ingredients in the slow cooker.
2. Cook on "high" for 4 hrs. Serve

Nutrition Info:

(Estimated Amount Per Serving): 343 Calories; 11 g Total Fat; 123 mg Cholesterol; 308 mg Sodium; 9 mg Carbohydrates; 3 g Dietary Fiber; 29 g Protein

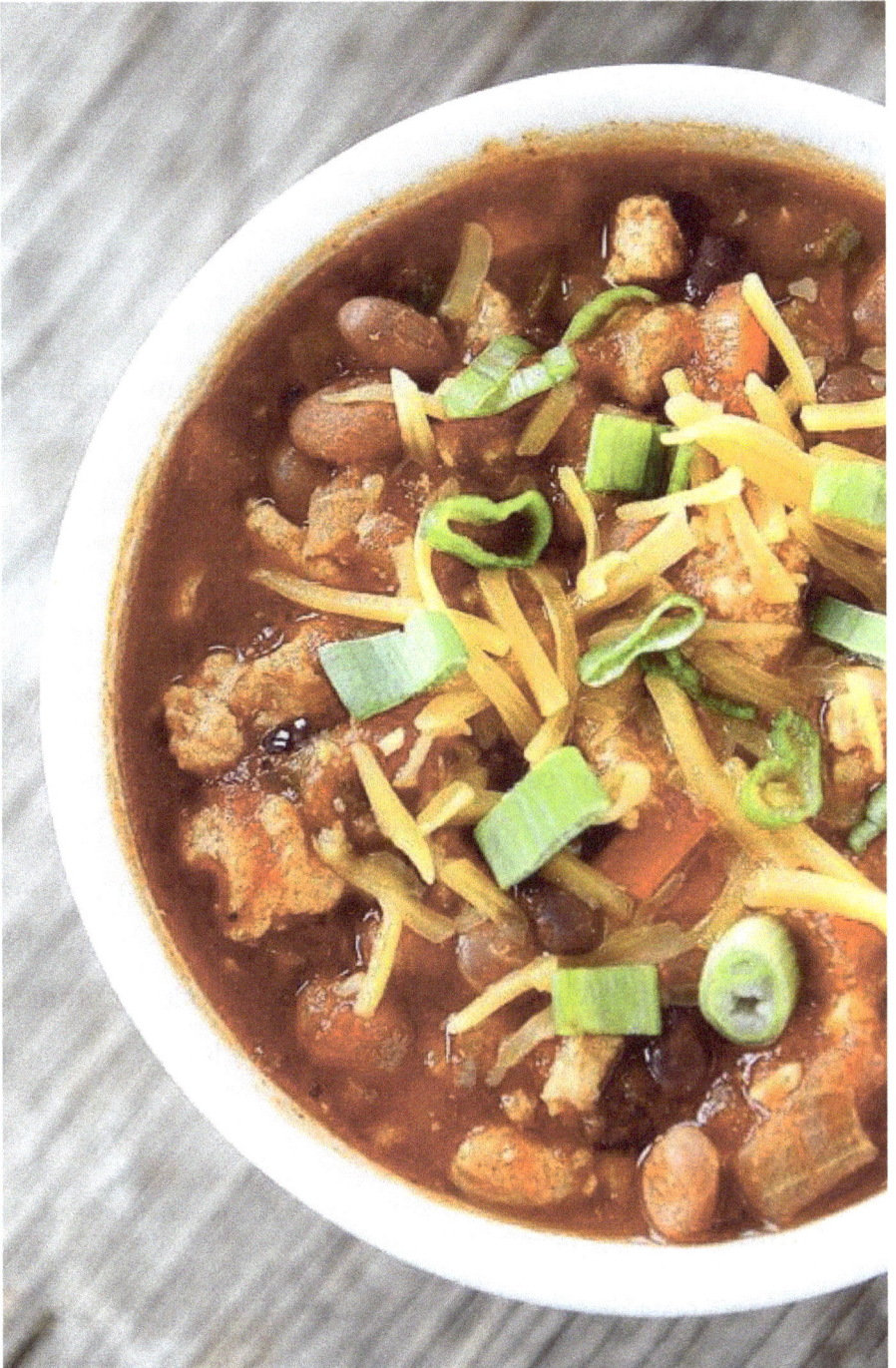

Broccoli Casserole

Servings: 6 Servings

Ingredients:

- 20 ounces (560 g) frozen broccoli spears
- 1 can (10 ounces, or 280 g) low-sodium cream of celery soup
- 1¼ cups (150 g) grated Cheddar cheese, divided
- ¼ cup (25 g) minced scallions
- 12 saltines, crushed

Directions:

1. Spray slow cooker with nonstick cooking spray. In large bowl, combine broccoli, soup, 1 cup (115 g) of grated cheese, and scallions. Pour into prepared slow cooker. Sprinkle with crushed crackers and the remaining cheese. Cover and slip a wooden toothpick between lid and pot to vent. Cook on low 5 to 6 hours or on high 2 to 3 hours.

Nutrition Info:

Per serving: 190 g water; 220 calories (47% from fat, 20% from protein, 33% from carb); 11 g protein; 12 g total fat; 6 g saturated fat; 3 g monounsaturated fat; 1 g polyunsaturated fat; 19 g carb; 3 g fiber; 2 g sugar; 231 mg phosphorus; 264 mg calcium; 2 mg iron; 607 mg sodium; 398 mg potassium; 1030 IU vitamin A; 91 mg ATE vitamin E; 85 mg vitamin C; 35 mg cholesterol

Slow Cooker Lasagna

Servings: 8 Servings

Ingredients:

- 58 ounces (1.6 kg) low-sodium spaghetti sauce
- 8 ounces (225 g) uncooked lasagna noodles
- 4 cups (460 g) shredded mozzarella cheese
- 1¼ cups (280 g) fat-free cottage cheese

Directions:

1. Spray the interior of the cooker with nonstick cooking spray. Spread one-fourth of the sauce on the bottom of the slow cooker. Arrange one-third of the uncooked noodles over the sauce. Break to fit if necessary. Combine the cheeses in a bowl. Spoon one-third of the cheeses over the noodles. Repeat these layers twice. Top with remaining sauce. Cover and cook on low 4 hours.

Nutrition Info:

Per serving: 212 g water; 523 calories (39% from fat, 18% from protein, 42% from carb); 24 g protein; 23 g total fat; 9 g saturated fat; 11 g monounsaturated fat; 2 g polyunsaturated fat; 56 g carb;

7 g fiber; 25 g sugar; 320 mg phosphorus; 367 mg calcium; 3 mg iron; 471 mg sodium; 908 mg potassium; 1655 IU vitamin A; 101 mg ATE vitamin E; 23 mg vitamin C; 46 mg cholesterol

Brussels Sprouts Casserole

Servings: 3

Cooking Time: 4 Hrs 15 Mins

Ingredients:

- ¾ lb. Brussels Sprouts
- 1 diced slice Pancetta
- 1 minced clove Garlic
- 1 tbsp. chopped Shallot
- ¼ cup pine nuts (toasted)
- ¼ tsp. Black Pepper (cracked)
- 4 tbsp. Water

Directions:

1. Slice sprouts and place them in the slow cooker along with the water.
2. Cook on "high" for 1 hr.
3. Drain well.
4. Remove the fat from Pancetta.
5. Sauté the pancetta for 4 mins.
6. Add the shallots, garlic and 1/8 cup of Pine Nuts to the sauté.
7. Now, add the sprouts.Cook for 3 mins.

8. Transfer the prepared mixture to the slow cooker. Add black pepper. 4 tbsp. of water and cook again on "low" for 2 hrs.

9. Serve immediately.

Nutrition Info:

(Estimated Amount Per Serving): 128 Calories; 9 g Total Fats; 56 mg Sodium; 2 mg Cholesterol; 5 g Carbohydrates; 4 g Dietary Fiber; 5 g Protein

Pasta And Mushrooms

Servings: 4 Servings

Ingredients:

- 8 ounces (225 g) mushrooms, sliced
- ½ teaspoon minced garlic
- ¼ cup (14 g) chopped sun dried tomatoes
- ½ cup (120 ml) dry white wine
- ½ cup (120 ml) vegetable broth
- ¼ cup (15 g) chopped Italian parsley
- 1 pound (455 g) pasta

Directions:

1. Combine all ingredients except the pasta in the slow cooker, cover, and cook on low 4 to 6 hours. Cook pasta according to directions on box and serve with sauce.

Nutrition Info:

Per serving: 126 g water; 487 calories (7% from fat, 15% from protein, 78% from carb); 17 g protein; 4 g total fat; 1 g saturated fat; 1 g monounsaturated fat; 1 g polyunsaturated fat; 91 g carb; 5 g fiber; 4 g sugar; 287 mg phosphorus; 41 mg calcium; 2 mg iron;

49 mg sodium; 596 mg potassium; 405 IU vitamin A; 0 mg ATE vitamin E; 14 mg vitamin C; 0 mg cholesterol

Onion Cabbage

Servings: 4

Cooking Time: 6 Hours

Ingredients:

- 1 onion, sliced
- 1 cabbage, shredded
- 2 apples, peeled, cored and roughly chopped
- 3 tablespoons mustard
- 1 tablespoon olive oil
- 1 cup low-sodium chicken stock
- Black pepper to the taste

Directions:

1. Grease your slow cooker with the oil and add apples, cabbage and onions.
2. In a bowl, mix stock with mustard and black pepper, whisk well, pour this into your slow cooker, cover, cook on Low for 6 hours, divide between plates and serve as a side dish.

Nutrition Info:

Calories 148, Fat 6.5g, Cholesterol 0mg, Sodium 93mg, Carbohydrate 22.1g, Fiber 4.7g, Sugars 14g, Protein 3.1g, Potassium 227mg

Cheese Broccoli

Servings: 10

Cooking Time: 3 Hours

Ingredients:

- 10 ounces coconut cream
- 6 cups broccoli florets, chopped
- 1 and ½ cups low-fat cheese, shredded
- 2 tablespoons olive oil
- ¼ cup yellow onion, chopped

Directions:

1. Add the oil to your slow cooker, add broccoli, onion, coconut cream, sprinkle cheese, cover and cook on High for 3 hours.
2. Divide between plates and serve as a side dish.

Nutrition Info:

Calories 177, Fat 15.4g, Cholesterol 18mg, Sodium 128mg, Carbohydrate 5.7g, Fiber 2.1g, Sugars 2.1g, Protein 6.4g, Potassium 268mg

Mixed Squash Casserole

Servings: 8 Servings

Ingredients:

- 1½ cups (180 g) sliced zucchini
- 1½ cups (180 g) sliced yellow squash
- 1 cup (180 g) peeled and chopped tomatoes
- ¼ cup (25 g) sliced scallions
- ½ cup (75 g) chopped green bell pepper
- ¼ cup (60 ml) low-sodium chicken broth
- ¼ cup (30 g) bread crumbs

Directions:

1. In slow cooker, layer half the zucchini, squash, tomatoes, scallions, and green pepper. Repeat layers. Pour broth over vegetables. Sprinkle bread crumbs over top. Cover and cook on low 4 to 6 hours.

Nutrition Info:

Per serving: 79 g water; 28 calories (11% from fat, 17% from protein, 72% from carb); 1 g protein; 0 g total fat; 0 g saturated fat; 0 g monounsaturated fat; 0 g polyunsaturated fat; 5 g carb; 1 g fiber; 1 g sugar; 31 mg phosphorus; 17 mg calcium; 0 mg iron;

10 mg sodium; 192 mg potassium; 271 IU vitamin A; 0 mg ATE vitamin E; 20 mg vitamin C; 0 mg cholesterol

Mushroom Pasta Sauce

Servings: 8 Servings

Ingredients:

- 1 tablespoon (15 ml) olive oil 8
- ounces (225 g) mushrooms, sliced
- 1 cup (160 g) chopped onion
- 1 teaspoon minced garlic
- ½ teaspoon oregano
- ¼ cup (25 g) grated Parmesan cheese
- 1 can (6 ounces, or 170 g) no-salt-added tomato paste
- 24 ounces (680 g) no-salt-added tomato sauce

Directions:

1. Heat oil in a large skillet and sauté mushrooms, onion, and garlic until onions are transparent. Add to slow cooker. Add remaining ingredients to cooker. Mix well. Cover and cook on low 6 hours.

Nutrition Info:

Per serving: 136 g water; 92 calories (27% from fat, 18% from protein, 55% from carb); 4 g protein; 3 g total fat; 1 g saturated fat; 2 g monounsaturated fat; 0 g polyunsaturated fat; 13 g carb;

3 g fiber; 8 g sugar; 98 mg phosphorus; 61 mg calcium; 2 mg iron; 80 mg sodium; 657 mg potassium; 638 IU vitamin A; 4 mg ATE vitamin E; 18 mg vitamin C; 3 mg cholesterol

Garlic Cauliflower Puree

Servings: 6

Cooking Time: 5 Hours

Ingredients:

- 1/3 cup dill, chopped
- 1 cauliflower head, florets separated
- 6 garlic cloves
- A pinch of black pepper
- 2 tablespoons olive oil

Directions:

1. Put cauliflower in your slow cooker, add dill, garlic and water to cover them, cover, cook on High for 5 hours, drain, add pepper and oil, mash using a potato masher, whisk well and serve as a side dish.

Nutrition Info:

Calories 62, Fat 4.9g, Cholesterol 0mg, Sodium 19mg, Carbohydrate 4.8g, Fiber 1.5g, Sugars 1.1g, Protein 1.6g, Potassium 234mg

Vegetable Medley

Servings: 6 Servings

Ingredients:

- ¾ cup (120 g) sliced onion
- 1 cup (100 g) celery, cut in 2-inch (5 cm) strips
- 1 cup (130 g) carrots, cut in 2-inch (5 cm) strips
- 1 cup (100 g) green beans
- ½ cup (75 g) diced green bell pepper
- 1 large tomato, sliced
- ¼ cup (55 g) unsalted butter
- 1/8 teaspoon black pepper
- 1 tablespoon (13 g) sugar
- 3 tablespoons (25 g) tapioca

Directions:

1. Mix ingredients and place in slow cooker. Cook on
2. low for 3 to 4 hours.

Nutrition Info:

Per serving: 107 g water; 126 calories (54% from fat, 4% from protein, 42% from carb); 1 g protein; 8 g total fat; 5 g saturated fat; 2 g monounsaturated fat; 0 g polyunsaturated fat; 14 g carb;

2 g fiber; 5 g sugar; 35 mg phosphorus; 31 mg calcium; 1 mg iron; 34 mg sodium; 260 mg potassium; 4226 IU vitamin A; 63 mg ATE vitamin E; 23 mg vitamin C; 20 mg cholesterol

Lemon And Green Beans Salad

Servings: 4

Cooking Time: 3 Hours

Ingredients:

- 1 pound green beans, trimmed and halved
- 2 teaspoons avocado oil
- 1 cup low-sodium veggie stock
- 2 garlic cloves, minced
- Zest of 1 lemon, grated
- 1 teaspoon hot paprika
- Juice of 1 lemon

Directions:

1. In your slow cooker, combine the green beans with the oil, stock and the other ingredients, put the lid on and cook on Low for 3 hours.
2. Divide between plates and serve as a side dish.

Nutrition Info:

Calories 48, Fat 0.6g, Cholesterol 0mg, Sodium 77mg, Carbohydrate 9.6g, Fiber 4.1g, Sugars 2.2g, Protein 2.3g, Potassium 265mg

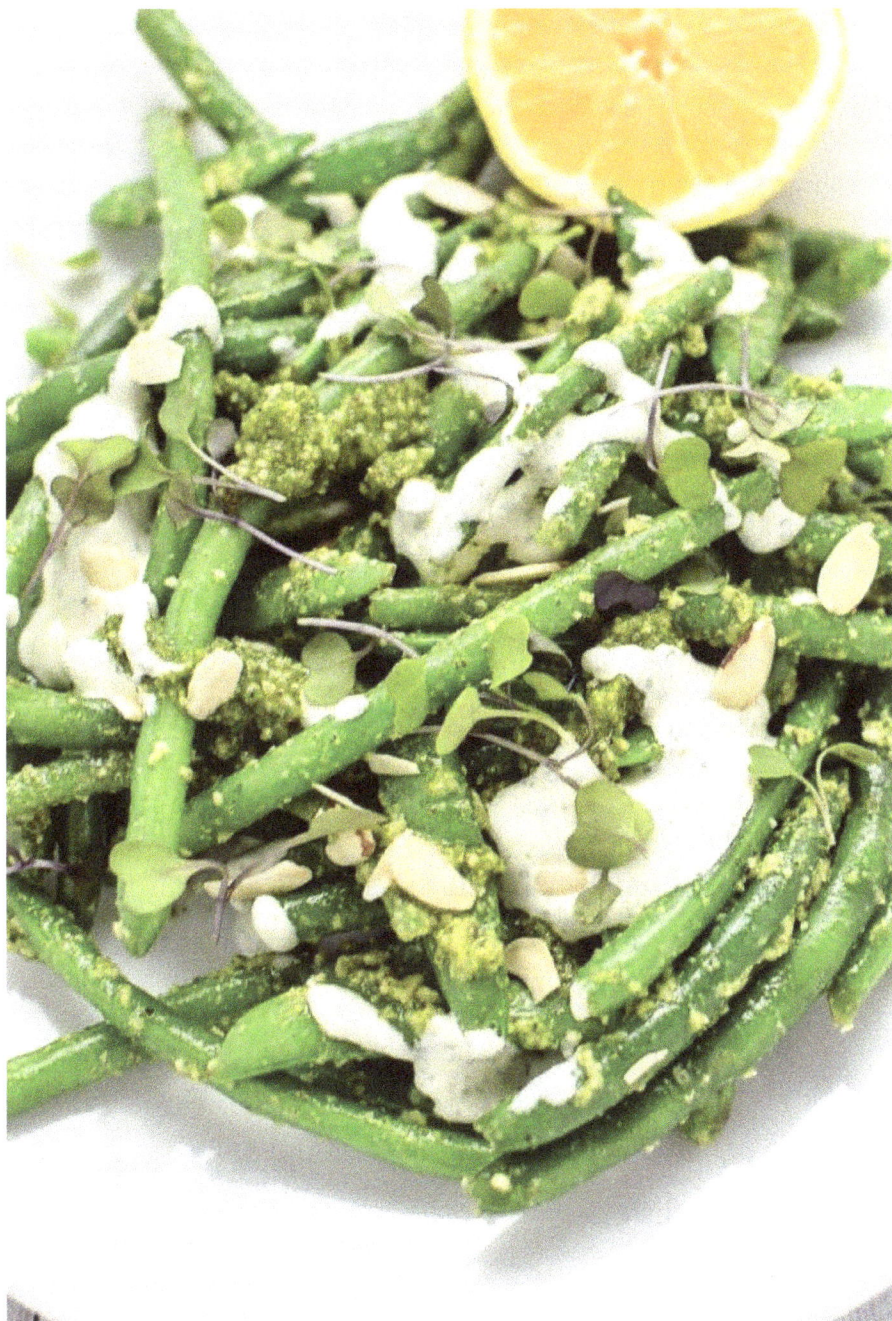

Tomatoes And Kale Side Dish

Servings: 6

Cooking Time: 2 Hours

Ingredients:

- 1 pound kale, chopped
- 2 teaspoons olive oil
- 1 tablespoons lemon juice
- 4 garlic cloves, minced
- ½ cup low-sodium veggie stock
- 1 cup cherry tomatoes, halved
- Black pepper to the taste

Directions:

1. Heat up a pan with the oil over medium heat, add garlic, stir, cook for 2 minutes and transfer to your slow cooker.
2. Add kale, stock, tomatoes, black pepper and lemon juice, cover, cook on High for 2 hours.
3. Divide the whole mix between plates and serve as a side dish.

Nutrition Info:

Calories 65, Fat 1.9g, Cholesterol 8mg, Sodium 84mg, Carbohydrate 10.5g, Fiber 1.6g, Sugars 1.2g, Protein 2.7g, Potassium 453mg

Spinach Casserole

Servings: 6 Servings

Ingredients:

- 20 ounces (560 g) frozen spinach, thawed and drained
- 2 cups (450 g) fat-free cottage cheese
- ½ cup (112 g) unsalted butter, cut into pieces
- 1½ cups (173 g) cubed Cheddar cheese
- ¾ cup (175 ml) egg substitute
- ¼ cup (31 g) flour

Directions:

1. Spray slow cooker with nonstick cooking spray. Combine all ingredients in a bowl and pour into prepared slow cooker. Cover and cook on low for 4 to 5 hours.

Nutrition Info:

Per serving: 188 g water; 398 calories (63% from fat, 25% from protein, 11% from carb); 26 g protein; 29 g total fat; 17 g saturated fat; 8 g monounsaturated fat; 2 g polyunsaturated fat; 12 g carb; 4 g fiber; 3 g sugar; 365 mg phosphorus; 450 mg calcium; 3 mg

iron; 474 mg sodium; 496 mg potassium; 12345 IU vitamin A; 220 mg ATE vitamin E; 2 mg vitamin C; 79 mg cholesterol

Thyme And Coconut Cauliflower Rice

Servings: 8

Cooking Time: 3 Hours

Ingredients:

- 3 cups low-sodium veggie stock
- 20 ounces spinach, chopped
- 2 garlic cloves, minced
- 6 ounces coconut cream
- 2 cups cauliflower rice
- 1 yellow onion, chopped
- ¼ teaspoon thyme, dried
- A pinch of black pepper
- 2 tablespoons olive oil

Directions:

1. Heat up a pan with the oil over medium heat, add onion, garlic, thyme and stock, stir, cook for 5 minutes and transfer to your slow cooker.

2. Add spinach, coconut cream, cauliflower rice and pepper, cover, cook on High for 3 hours, divide between plates and serve as a side dish.

Nutrition Info:

Calories 122, Fat 9.3g, Cholesterol 0mg, Sodium 116mg, Carbohydrate 7.4g, Fiber 2.4g, Sugars 2.6g, Protein 4.5g, Potassium 475mg

Spiced Broccoli Florets

Servings: 10

Cooking Time: 3 Hours

Ingredients:

- 6 cups broccoli florets
- 1 and ½ cups low-fat cheddar cheese, shredded
- ½ teaspoon cider vinegar
- ¼ cup yellow onion, chopped
- 10 ounces tomato sauce, sodium-free
- 2 tablespoons olive oil
- A pinch of black pepper

Directions:

1. Grease your slow cooker with the oil, add broccoli, tomato sauce, cider vinegar, onion and black pepper, cover and cook on High for 2 hours and 30 minutes.
2. Sprinkle the cheese all over, cover, cook on High for 30 minutes more, divide between plates and serve as a side dish.

Nutrition Info:

Calories 119, Fat 8.7g, Cholesterol 18mg, Sodium 272mg, Carbohydrate 5.7g, Fiber 1.9g, Sugars 2.3g, Protein 6.2g, Potassium 288mg

Apple Salsa

Servings: 3

Cooking Time: 2 Hrs

Ingredients:

- 7 ½ oz. drained Black Beans
- ¼ cubed Apples (Granny Smith)
- ¼ chopped Chili Pepper (Serrano)
- 1/8 cup chopped Onion (red)
- 1 ½ tbsp. chopped Cilantro
- ¼ Lemon
- ¼ Orange
- Pinch of Sea Salt
- Pinch of Black Pepper (cracked)

Directions:

1. Mix all the ingredients in the cooker (slow cooker).
2. Cook on "low" for an hour.
3. Transfer to a covered container and allow to cool for 1 hr.
4. Serve.

Nutrition Info:

(Estimated Amount Per Serving): 100 Calories; 0.4 g Total Fats; 50 mg Sodium; 0 mg Cholesterol; 20 g Carbohydrates; 6 g Dietary Fiber; 5 g Protein

Onion And Eggplant Salad

Servings: 6

Cooking Time: 2 Hours

Ingredients:

- 14 ounces canned roasted tomatoes, no-salt-added and chopped
- 4 cups kale, torn
- 4 cups eggplant, cubed
- 1 yellow bell pepper, chopped
- 1 red onion, cut into medium wedges
- 3 tablespoons red vinegar
- 1 garlic clove, minced
- 2 tablespoons olive oil
- 1 teaspoon mustard
- ½ cup parsley, chopped
- A pinch of black pepper

Directions:

1. In your slow cooker, mix eggplant with tomatoes, bell pepper and onion, cover and cook on High for 2 hours.
2. In a bowl, mix oil with vinegar, mustard, garlic and pepper, whisk well, add to your slow cooker, also add

kale and parsley, toss, divide between plates and serve as a side dish.

Nutrition Info:

Calories 103, Fat 5g, Cholesterol 0mg, Sodium 175mg, Carbohydrate 14.8g, Fiber 4.2g, Sugars 4.3g, Protein 2.9g, Potassium 556mg

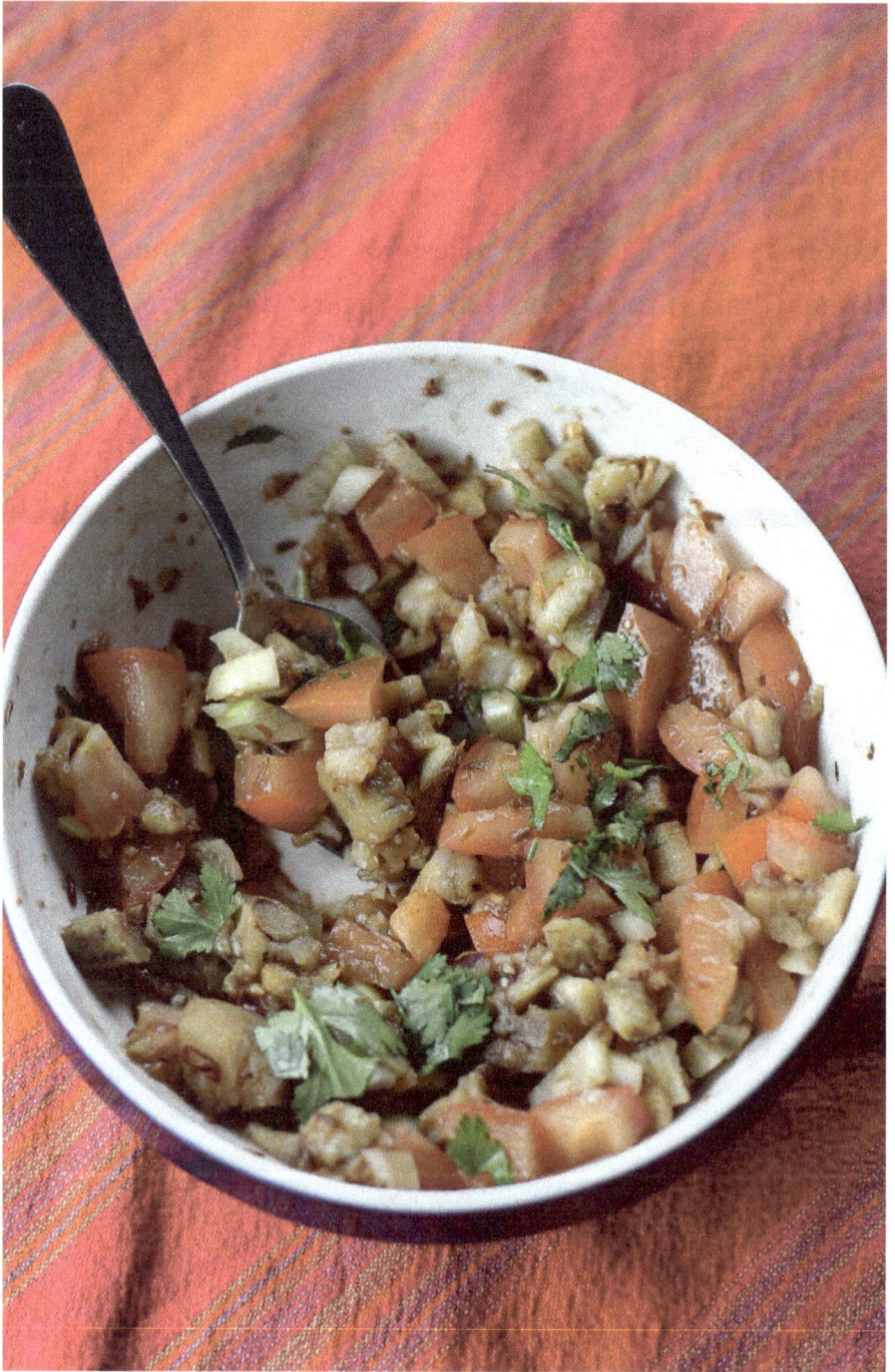

Cream Cheese Rice

Servings: 8

Cooking Time: 4 Hours

Ingredients:

- 20 ounces spinach, chopped
- 8 ounces fat-free cream cheese
- 2 tablespoons olive oil
- 2 cups wild rice
- 2 cups low-fat cheddar cheese, shredded
- 1 yellow onion, chopped
- ¼ teaspoon thyme, dried
- 2 garlic cloves, minced
- 4 cups low-sodium chicken stock
- ½ cup whole wheat bread, crumbled

Directions:

1. In your slow cooker, mix the oil with the onion, thyme, garlic, stock, spinach, cream cheese and rice, toss, cover and cook on Low for 4 hours.
2. Add the cheese and the breadcrumbs, cover the pot, leave it aside for a few minutes, divide between plates and serve as a side dish.

Nutrition Info:

Calories 448, Fat 24g, Cholesterol 61mg, Sodium 460mg, Carbohydrate 41.4g, Fiber 5.4g, Sugars 2.9g, Protein 19.7g, Potassium 688mg

Vegetarian Spaghetti Sauce

Servings: 6 Servings

Ingredients:

- 4 cups (328 g) eggplant, peeled and cut into 1-inch (2.5 cm) cubes
- 1 cup (160 g) chopped onion
- 2 cups (300 g) chopped red bell pepper
- 4 teaspoons (12 g) minced garlic
- 1 can (28 ounces, or 785 g) no-salt-added crushed tomatoes, undrained
- 1 can (28 ounces, or 785 g) no-salt-added diced tomatoes, undrained
- 1 can (6 ounces, or 170 g) no-salt-added tomato paste
- 2 tablespoons (30 g) brown sugar
- 2 tablespoons (12 g) Italian seasoning
- ¼ teaspoon red pepper flakes

Directions:

1. In a slow cooker, combine all ingredients. Cover and cook on low for 10 to 12 hours or on high for 5 to 6 hours.

Nutrition Info:

Per serving: 392 g water; 128 calories (5% from fat, 13% from protein, 82% from carb); 5 g protein; 1 g total fat; 0 g saturated fat; 0 g monounsaturated fat; 0 g polyunsaturated fat; 30 g carb; 8 g fiber; 19 g sugar; 114 mg phosphorus; 130 mg calcium; 4 mg iron; 69 mg sodium; 1096 mg potassium; 2412 IU vitamin A; 0 mg ATE vitamin E; 99 mg vitamin C; 0 mg cholesterol

Greek Stuffed Peppers

Servings: 4 Servings

Ingredients:

- 4 green bell peppers
- ½ cup (120 ml) vegetable broth, boiling
- ½ cup (88 g) couscous
- 2 teaspoons white wine vinegar
- 3 ounces (85 g) feta cheese, crumbled
- 3 tablespoons (27 g) pine nuts
- 1 tablespoon (1.3 g) dried parsley
- ¼ teaspoon freshly ground black pepper

Directions:

1. Halve the peppers and remove the seeds; set aside. Pour the boiling broth over the couscous, cover, and let stand 5 minutes. Fluff with a fork and then stir in the remaining ingredients. Stuff couscous mixture into the peppers and then place peppers in the bottom of the slow cooker. Turn to high, pour 2/3 cup (160 ml) of boiling water around the peppers, cover, and cook until peppers are tender, about 2 hours.

Nutrition Info:

Per serving: 186 g water; 224 calories (39% from fat, 14% from protein, 47% from carb); 8 g protein; 10 g total fat; 4 g saturated fat; 3 g monounsaturated fat; 3 g polyunsaturated fat; 27 g carb; 4 g fiber; 5 g sugar; 182 mg phosphorus; 132 mg calcium; 1 mg iron; 262 mg sodium; 368 mg potassium; 723 IU vitamin A; 27 mg ATE vitamin E; 122 mg vitamin C; 19 mg cholesterol

Parmesan Artichokes

Servings: 8

Cooking Time: 5 Hours

Ingredients:

- 4 artichokes, trimmed and halved
- 2 cups whole wheat breadcrumbs
- 1 cup low-sodium vegetable stock
- Juice of 1 lemon
- 3 garlic cloves, minced
- 1 tablespoon lemon zest, grated
- 2 tablespoons parsley, chopped
- 1/3 cup low-fat parmesan, grated
- Black pepper to the taste
- 1 tablespoon olive oil
- 1 tablespoon shallot, minced
- 1 teaspoon oregano, chopped

Directions:

1. Rub artichokes with the lemon juice and the oil and put them in your slow cooker.

2. Add breadcrumbs, garlic, parsley, parmesan, lemon zest, black pepper, shallot, oregano and stock, cover and cook on Low for 5 hours.

3. Divide the whole mix between plates, sprinkle parsley on top and serve as a side dish.

Nutrition Info:

Calories 149, Fat 2.8g, Cholesterol 1mg, Sodium 188mg, Carbohydrate 26g, Fiber 6.7g, Sugars 2.1g, Protein 7.7g, Potassium 368mg

Mexi-corn

Servings: 8 Servings

Ingredients:

- 20 ounces (580 g) frozen corn, partially thawed
- 4 ounces (115 g) pimientos, chopped
- ¼ cup (38 g) finely chopped green bell pepper
- ¼ cup (60 ml) water
- ¼ teaspoon pepper
- ½ teaspoon paprika
- ½ teaspoon chili powder

Directions:

1. Combine all ingredients in slow cooker. Cover and cook on high 45 minutes, then on low 2 to 4 hours. Stir occasionally.

Nutrition Info:

Per serving: 79 g water; 62 calories (5% from fat, 12% from protein, 83% from carb); 2 g protein; 0 g total fat; 0 g saturated fat; 0 g monounsaturated fat; 0 g polyunsaturated fat; 15 g carb; 2 g fiber; 3 g sugar; 45 mg phosphorus; 5 mg calcium; 1 mg iron;

8 mg sodium; 141 mg potassium; 521 IU vitamin A; 0 mg ATE vitamin E; 18 mg vitamin C; 0 mg cholesterol

Lemon Asparagus

Servings: 4

Cooking Time: 2 Hours

Ingredients:

- 1 pound asparagus, trimmed and halved
- 1 tablespoon parsley, chopped
- ¼ teaspoon lemon zest, grated
- 2 teaspoons lemon juice
- ½ cup low-sodium veggie stock
- 1 garlic clove, minced

Directions:

1. In your slow cooker, mix the asparagus with the parsley, stock, garlic, lemon zest and lemon juice, toss a bit, cover and cook on High for 2 hours.
2. Divide the asparagus between plates and serve as a side dish.

Nutrition Info:

Calories 27, Fat 0.2g, Cholesterol 0mg, Sodium 21mg, Carbohydrate 5g, Fiber 2.5g, Sugars 2.3g, Protein 2.6g, Potassium 241mg

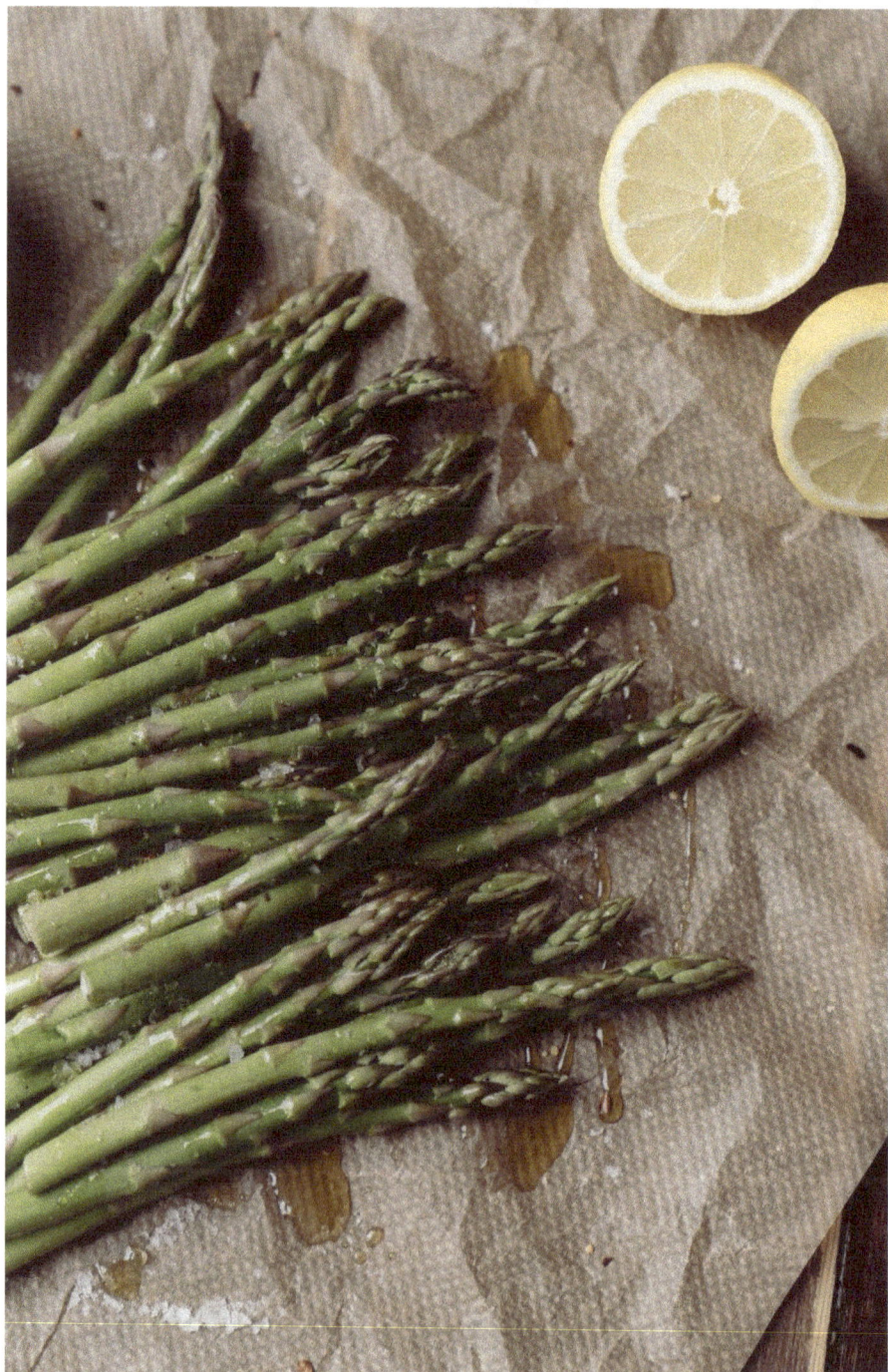

Tender Swiss Chard

Servings: 4

Cooking Time: 2 Hours

Ingredients:

- 2 tablespoons olive oil
- 2 bunches Swiss chard, roughly torn
- 3 tablespoons lemon juice
- ½ cup low-sodium veggie stock
- Black pepper to the taste
- ½ teaspoon garlic paste

Directions:

1. In your slow cooker, mix oil with chard, stock, lemon juice, garlic paste and pepper, toss, cover, cook on High for 2 hours, divide between plates and serve.

Nutrition Info:

Calories 75, Fat 7.4g, Cholesterol 0mg, Sodium 106mg, Carbohydrate 2g, Fiber 0.4g, Sugars 0.9g, Protein 0.7g, Potassium 84mg

Creamed Spinach

Servings: 8 Servings

Ingredients:

- 30 ounces (840 g) frozen spinach
- 2 cups (450 g) fat-free cottage cheese
- 1 cup (115 g) shredded Cheddar
- ¾ cup (175 ml) egg substitute
- ¼ cup (30 g) flour
- ½ cup (112 g) unsalted butter, melted

Directions:

1. Mix together all ingredients and pour into slow cooker. Cook on high for 1 hour, then on low for 4 hours more.

Nutrition Info:

Per serving: 170 g water; 277 calories (59% from fat, 26% from protein, 14% from carb); 19 g protein; 19 g total fat; 11 g saturated fat; 5 g monounsaturated fat; 1 g polyunsaturated fat; 10 g carb; 4 g fiber; 2 g sugar; 249 mg phosphorus; 333 mg calcium; 3 mg iron; 339 mg sodium; 471 mg potassium; 13450 IU vitamin A; 144 mg ATE vitamin E; 2 mg vitamin C; 50 mg cholesterol

Lentils And Rice

Servings: 8 Servings

Ingredients:

- 1½ cups (240 g) sliced onions
- 2 tablespoons (28 ml) olive oil
- 6 cups (1.4 L) water
- 1 cup (192 g) lentils, sorted, washed, and drained
- 2 cups (380 g) brown rice, washed and drained

Directions:

1. Place onions in nonstick skillet with olive oil. Sauté over medium heat until onions are golden brown. Remove about ½ cup (80 g) from skillet and place on paper towel to drain. Place remaining onions and drippings in slow cooker. Combine with water, lentils, and brown rice. Cover and cook on low 6 to 8 hours. Garnish with reserved onions.

Nutrition Info:

Per serving: 257 g water; 125 calories (28% from fat, 12% from protein, 60% from carb); 4 g protein; 4 g total fat; 1 g saturated fat; 3 g monounsaturated fat; 1 g polyunsaturated fat; 19 g carb; 3

g fiber; 2 g sugar; 94 mg phosphorus; 22 mg calcium; 1 mg iron; 10 mg sodium; 158 mg potassium; 3 IU vitamin A; 0 mg ATE vitamin E; 3 mg vitamin C; 0 mg cholesterol

Mushroom Lasagna

Servings: 8 Servings

Ingredients:

- 6 ounces (170 g) uncooked lasagna noodles
- 28 ounces (785 g) low-sodium spaghetti sauce
- 1/3 cup (80 ml) water
- 8 ounces (225 g) mushrooms, sliced
- 15 ounces (425 g) ricotta cheese
- 2 cups (230 g) shredded mozzarella cheese

Directions:

1. Break noodles. Place half in bottom of greased slow cooker. Layer half of sauce and water, half of mushrooms, half of ricotta cheese, and half of mozzarella cheese over noodles. Repeat layers. Cover and cook on low 5 hours.

Nutrition Info:

Per serving: 164 g water; 351 calories (40% from fat, 20% from protein, 40% from carb); 18 g protein; 16 g total fat; 7 g saturated fat; 6 g monounsaturated fat; 1 g polyunsaturated fat; 36 g carb;

4 g fiber; 12 g sugar; 256 mg phosphorus; 319 mg calcium; 2 mg iron; 275 mg sodium; 593 mg potassium; 1003 IU vitamin A; 105

Greek Green Beans and Tomatoes

Servings: 4 Servings

Ingredients:

- 1 pound (455 g) fresh green beans, cut into 1-inch (2.5 cm) lengths
- ½ teaspoon crushed garlic
- 1 cup (235 ml) no-salt-added diced tomatoes
- 1 cup (160 g) chopped onion
- ½ teaspoon dried oregano
- 1 teaspoon lemon juice
- 1 tablespoon (15 ml) olive oil
- Black pepper, to taste

Directions:

1. Place ingredients in slow cooker. Stir. Cover and cook on low for 6 hours.

Nutrition Info:

Per serving: 193 g water; 92 calories (32% from fat, 12% from protein, 56% from carb); 3 g protein; 4 g total fat; 1 g saturated fat; 2 g monounsaturated fat; 0 g polyunsaturated fat; 14 g carb; 5 g fiber; 5 g sugar; 66 mg phosphorus; 71 mg calcium; 2 mg iron; 16 mg sodium; 407 mg potassium; 858 IU vitamin A; 0 mg ATE vitamin E; 27 mg vitamin C; 0 mg cholesterol

Pasta And Red Beans

Servings: 8 Servings

Ingredients:

- 5 cups (1.2 L) low-sodium vegetable broth
- 1 teaspoon cumin
- 1 tablespoon (7.5 g) chili powder
- ½ teaspoon minced garlic
- 8 ounces (225 g) uncooked pasta
- ½ cup (75 g) diced green bell pepper
- ½ cup (75 g) diced red bell pepper
- ¾ cup (120 g) diced onion
- 1 can (15 ounces, or 425 g) no-salt-added kidney beans, rinsed and drained

Directions:

1. Combine broth, cumin, chili powder, and garlic in slow cooker. Cover and cook on high until mixture comes to boil. Add pasta, vegetables, and beans. Stir together well. Cover and cook on low 3 to 4 hours.

Nutrition Info:

Per serving: 216 g water; 206 calories (7% from fat, 24% from protein, 70% from carb); 12 g protein; 2 g total fat; 0 g saturated fat; 0 g monounsaturated fat; 0 g polyunsaturated fat; 36 g carb; 6 g fiber; 2 g sugar; 185 mg phosphorus; 83 mg calcium; 2 mg iron; 94 mg sodium; 458 mg potassium; 337 IU vitamin A; 2 mg ATE vitamin E; 21 mg vitamin C; 0 mg cholesterol

Baby Spinach Mix

Servings: 6

Cooking Time: 4 Hours

Ingredients:

- 5 carrots, sliced
- 5 ounces baby spinach
- 1 yellow onion, chopped
- 1 and ½ cups great northern beans, dried
- 2 garlic cloves, minced
- 2 teaspoons lemon peel, grated
- 3 tablespoons lemon juice
- Black pepper to the taste
- ½ teaspoon oregano, dried
- 4 and ½ cups low-sodium veggie stock

Directions:

1. In your slow cooker, mix beans with onion, carrots, garlic, pepper, oregano and stock, stir, cover and cook on High for 4 hours.
2. Add spinach, lemon juice and lemon peel, stir, leave aside for 5 minutes, divide between plates and serve.

Nutrition Info:

Calories 208, Fat 0.9g, Cholesterol 0mg, Sodium 152mg, Carbohydrate 38.1g, Fiber 11.6g, Sugars 4.9g, Protein 13g, Potassium 973mg

Orange Beets

Servings: 8

Cooking Time: 6 Hours

Ingredients:

- 6 beets, peeled and sliced
- 1/3 cup orange juice
- 1 teaspoon orange peel, grated
- 2 tablespoons stevia
- 1 tablespoon ginger, grated
- A pinch of black pepper
- 2 tablespoons white vinegar
- 2 tablespoons olive oil

Directions:

1. In your slow cooker, mix the beets with the orange peel, orange juice, stevia, vinegar, oil, ginger and black pepper, toss, cover and cook on Low for 6 hours.
2. Divide between plates and serve as a side dish.

Nutrition Info:

Calories 71, Fat 3.7g, Cholesterol 0mg, Sodium 58mg, Carbohydrate 12.9g, Fiber 1.6g, Sugars 6.9g, Protein 1.4g, Potassium 262mg

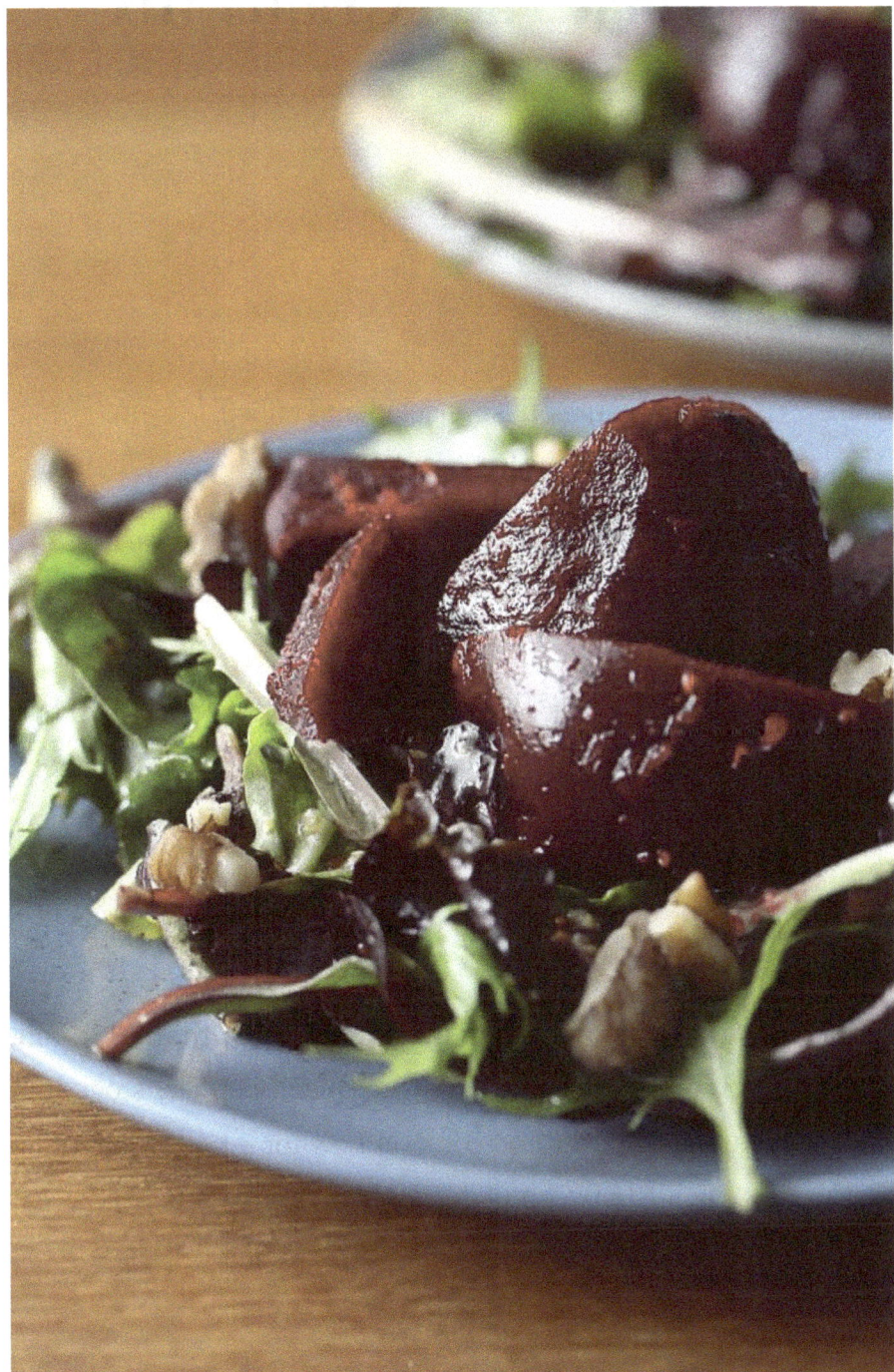

Baby Spinach and Grains Mix

Servings: 12

Cooking Time: 4 Hours

Ingredients:

- 1 butternut squash, peeled and cubed
- 1 cup whole grain blend, uncooked
- 12 ounces low-sodium veggie stock
- 6 ounces baby spinach
- 1 yellow onion, chopped
- 3 garlic cloves, minced
- ½ cup water
- 2 teaspoons thyme, chopped
- A pinch of black pepper

Directions:

1. In your slow cooker, mix the squash with whole grain, onion, garlic, water, thyme, black pepper, stock and spinach, cover and cook on Low for 4 hours.
2. Divide between plates and serve as a side dish.

Nutrition Info:

Calories78, Fat 0.6g, Cholesterol 0mg, Sodium 259mg, Carbohydrate 16.4g, Fiber 1.8g, Sugars 2g, Protein 2.5g, Potassium 138mg

Tomato Sauce Green Beans

Servings: 10

Cooking Time: 2 Hours

Ingredients:

- 16 cups green beans, halved
- ½ cup coconut sugar
- ¼ cup tomato sauce, no-salt-added
- ¾ teaspoon low sodium soy sauce
- 3 tablespoons olive oil
- A pinch of black pepper

Directions:

1. In your slow cooker, mix green beans with coconut sugar, tomato sauce, pepper, soy sauce and oil, cover and cook on Low for 3 hours.
2. Divide between plates and serve as a side dish.

Nutrition Info:

Calories 98, Fat 4.4g, Cholesterol 0mg, Sodium 58mg, Carbohydrate 13.9g, Fiber 6.1g, Sugars 2.7g, Protein 3.4g, Potassium 389mg

Lentil Sauce

Servings: 6 Servings

Ingredients:

- ½ cup (80 g) chopped onion
- ¼ cup (33 g) chopped carrots
- ¼ cup (25 g) chopped celery
- 2 cups (480 ml) diced tomatoes
- 1 can (8 ounces, or 225 g) no-salt-added tomato sauce
- ½ cup (96 g) lentils, rinsed and drained
- ½ teaspoon oregano
- ¼ teaspoon basil
- ¼ teaspoon garlic powder
- ¼ teaspoon red pepper flakes

Directions:

1. Mix all ingredients in slow cooker. Cover and cook on low 8 to 10 hours or on high 3 to 5 hours.

Nutrition Info:

Per serving: 112 g water; 57 calories (6% from fat, 19% from protein, 75% from carb); 3 g protein; 0 g total fat; 0 g saturated fat; 0 g monounsaturated fat; 0 g polyunsaturated fat; 11 g carb;

4 g fiber; 3 g sugar; 69 mg phosphorus; 53 mg calcium; 2 mg iron; 17 mg sodium; 419 mg potassium; 1547 IU vitamin A; 0 mg ATE vitamin E; 21 mg vitamin C; 0 mg cholesterol

Chickpeas And Curried Veggies

Servings: About 2

Cooking Time: 4 Hrs

Ingredients:

- ½ tbsp. Canola Oil
- 2 sliced Celery Ribs
- 1/8 tsp. Cayenne Pepper
- ¼ cup Water
- 2 sliced Carrots
- 2 sliced red Potatoes (sliced)
- ½ tbsp. Curry Powder
- ½ cup o Coconut Milk (light)
- ¼ cup drained Chickpeas (low sodium)
- Chopped Cilantro
- ¼ cup Yogurt (low fat)

Directions:

1. Sauté potatoes for 5 mins in oil.
2. Add the carrots, celery and onion.Sauté for 5 more mins.
3. Sprinkle on the curry powder and cayenne pepper.Stir well to combine.

4. In slow cooker, pour water and coconut milk.

5. Add in the potatoes.

6. Cook on "low" for 3 hrs.

7. Add chickpeas and cook for 30 more mins.

8. Serve in bowls along with the yogurt and cilantro garnish.

Nutrition Info:

(Estimated Amount Per Serving): 271 Calories; 11 g Total Fats; 2 mg Cholesterol; 207 mg Sodium; 39 g Carbohydrates; 8 g Dietary Fiber; 7 g Protein

Glazed Carrots

Servings: 8 Servings

Ingredients:

- 2 pounds (900 g) carrots, sliced
- ½ cup (80 g) chopped onion
- ¼ cup (60 ml) water
- ¼ cup (85 g) honey
- ¼ cup (80 g) apricot preserves

Directions:

1. Place carrots and onions in slow cooker. Add water. Cover and cook on low 9 hours. Drain liquid from slow cooker. In a small bowl, mix honey and preserves together. Pour over carrots. Cover and cook on high 10 to 15 minutes.

Nutrition Info:

Per serving: 121 g water; 110 calories (2% from fat, 4% from protein, 94% from carb); 1 g protein; 0 g total fat; 0 g saturated fat; 0 g monounsaturated fat; 0 g polyunsaturated fat; 27 g carb; 3 g fiber; 19 g sugar; 45 mg phosphorus; 43 mg calcium; 0 mg

iron; 82 mg sodium; 391 mg potassium; 19064 IU vitamin A; 0 mg ATE vitamin E; 8 mg vitamin C; 0 mg cholesterol

Squash Casserole

Servings: 6 Servings

Ingredients:

- 4 cups (480 g) thinly sliced yellow squash
- ½ cup (80 g) chopped onion
- 1 cup (130 g) shredded carrot
- 1 can (10 ounces, or 280 g) low-sodium cream of chicken soup
- 1 cup (230 g) fat-free sour cream
- ¼ cup (31 g) flour
- 8 ounces (225 g) reduced-sodium stuffing mix, crumbled
- ½ cup (112 g) unsalted butter, melted

Directions:

1. In large bowl, combine squash, onion, carrot, and soup. Mix sour cream and flour together; stir into vegetables. Toss stuffing crumbs with butter and place half in slow cooker. Add vegetable mixture and top with remaining stuffing crumbs. Cover and cook on low for 7 to 9 hours.

Nutrition Info:

Per serving: 182 g water; 426 calories (51% from fat, 8% from protein, 41% from carb); 9 g protein; 25 g total fat; 14 g saturated fat; 7 g monounsaturated fat; 2 g polyunsaturated fat; 44 g carb; 3 g fiber; 7 g sugar; 157 mg phosphorus; 112 mg calcium; 3 mg iron; 668 mg sodium; 465 mg potassium; 4453 IU vitamin A; 188 mg ATE vitamin E; 15 mg vitamin C; 61 mg cholesterol

Mushroom Sausages

Servings: 12

Cooking Time: 2 Hours

Ingredients:

- 6 celery ribs, chopped
- 1 pound no-sugar, beef sausage, chopped
- 2 tablespoons olive oil
- ½ pound mushrooms, chopped
- ½ cup sunflower seeds, peeled
- 1 cup low-sodium veggie stock
- 1 cup cranberries, dried
- 2 yellow onions, chopped
- 2 garlic cloves, minced
- 1 tablespoon sage, dried
- 1 whole wheat bread loaf, cubed

Directions:

1. Heat up a pan with the oil over medium- high heat, add beef, stir and brown for a few minutes.
2. Add mushrooms, onion, celery, garlic and sage, stir, cook for a few more minutes and transfer to your slow cooker.

3. Add stock, cranberries, sunflower seeds and the bread cubes, cover and cook on High for 2 hours.
4. Stir the whole mix, divide between plates and serve as a side dish.

Nutrition Info:

Calories 188, Fat 13.8g, Cholesterol 25mg, Sodium 489mg, Carbohydrate 8.2g, Fiber 1.9g, Sugars 2.2g, Protein 7.6g, Potassium 254mg

Lentil Meal

Servings: 8 Servings

Ingredients:

- 8 ounces (225 g) dried lentils, rinsed
- 2 cups (470 ml) water
- 1 whole bay leaf
- ¼ teaspoon pepper
- 1/8 teaspoon marjoram
- 1/8 teaspoon sage
- 1/8 teaspoon thyme
- 2 cups (320 g) chopped onions
- ½ teaspoon minced garlic
- 2 cups (300 g) canned no-salt-added diced tomatoes
- ½ cup (65 g) carrots, sliced 1/8 inch (32 mm) thick
- ½ cup (50 g) celery, thinly sliced 3 medium potatoes, diced
- ½ cup (75 g) chopped green bell pepper
- 2 tablespoons (8 g) finely chopped fresh parsley
- 1½ cups (173 g) shredded Cheddar cheese

Directions:

1. Mix all ingredients except cheese in slow cooker; cover and cook on high 6 hours. Remove bay leaf and add cheese just before serving.

Nutrition Info:

Per serving: 315 g water; 263 calories (29% from fat, 18% from protein, 53% from carb); 12 g protein; 9 g total fat; 5 g saturated fat; 2 g monounsaturated fat; 0 g polyunsaturated fat; 36 g carb; 6 g fiber; 6 g sugar; 292 mg phosphorus; 236 mg calcium; 3 mg iron; 185 mg sodium; 995 mg potassium; 1823 IU vitamin A; 64 mg ATE vitamin E; 30 mg vitamin C; 26 mg cholesterol

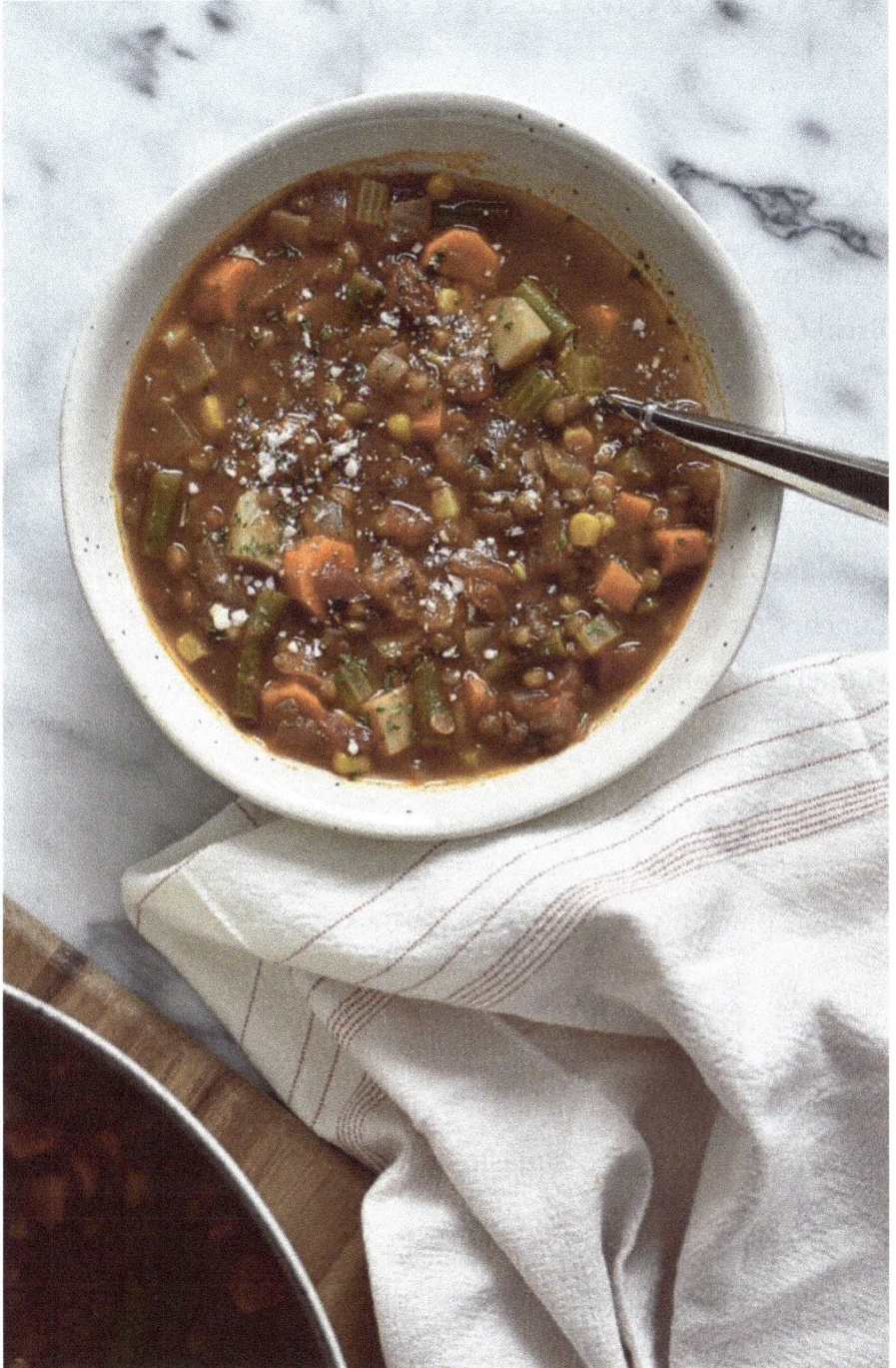

4-WEEK MEAL PLAN

Week 1

Monday
Breakfast: Tofu Frittata
Lunch: Pork Chops In Beer
Dinner: Stewed Tomatoes

Tuesday
Breakfast: Tapioca
Lunch: Creamy Beef Burgundy
Dinner: Oregano Salad

Wednesday
Breakfast: Fruit Oats
Lunch: Smothered Steak
Dinner: Black Beans With Corn Kernels

Thursday
Breakfast: Grapefruit Mix
Lunch: Pork For Sandwiches
Dinner: Stuffed Acorn Squash

Friday
Breakfast: Berry Yogurt
Lunch: Cranberry Pork Roast

Dinner: Greek Eggplant

Saturday
Breakfast: Soft Pudding
Lunch: Pan-asian Pot Roast
Dinner: Thyme Sweet Potatoes

Sunday
Breakfast: Black Beans Salad
Lunch: Short Ribs
Dinner: Barley Vegetable Soup

Week 2

Monday
Breakfast: Carrot Pudding
Lunch: French Dip
Dinner: Butter Corn

Tuesday
Breakfast: Apple Cake
Lunch: Italian Roast With Vegetables
Dinner: Orange Glazed Carrots

Wednesday
Breakfast: Almond Milk Barley Cereals
Lunch: Honey Mustard Ribs
Dinner: Cinnamon Acorn Squash

Thursday

Breakfast: Cashews Cake

Lunch: Pizza Casserole

Dinner: Glazed Root Vegetables

Friday

Breakfast: Artichoke Frittata

Lunch: Hawaiian Pork Roast

Dinner: Stir Fried Steak, Shiitake And Asparagus

Saturday

Breakfast: Mexican Eggs

Lunch: Apple Cranberry Pork Roast

Dinner: Cilantro Brussel Sprouts

Sunday

Breakfast: Stewed Peach

Lunch: Swiss Steak

Dinner: Italian Zucchini

Week 3

Monday

Breakfast: Lamb Cassoule t

Lunch: Glazed Pork Roast

Dinner: Cilantro Parsnip Chunks

Tuesday

Breakfast: Fruited Tapioca

Lunch: Swiss Steak In Wine Sauce

Dinner: Corn Casserole

Wednesday

Breakfast: Baby Spinach Shrimp Salad

Lunch: Italian Pork Chops

Dinner: Pilaf With Bella Mushrooms

Thursday

Breakfast: Coconut And Fruit Cake

Lunch: Italian Pot Roast

Dinner: Italian Style Yellow Squash

Friday

Breakfast: Apple And Squash Bowls

Lunch: Beef With Horseradish Sauce

Dinner: Stevia Peas With Marjoram

Saturday

Breakfast: Slow Cooker Chocolate Cake

Lunch: Oriental Pot Roast

Dinner: Broccoli Rice Casserole

Sunday

Breakfast: Fish Omelet

Lunch: Barbecued Ribs

Dinner: Italians Style Mushroom Mix

Week 4

Monday
Breakfast: Brown Cake
Lunch: Ham And Scalloped Pota toes
Dinner: Broccoli Casserole

Tuesday
Breakfast: Stevia And Walnuts Cut Oats
Lunch: Pork And Pineapple Roast

Wednesday
Breakfast: Walnut And Cinnamon Oatmeal
Lunch: Barbecued Brisket
Dinner: Dinner: Slow Cooker Lasagna

Thursday
Breakfast: Tender Rosemary Sweet Potatoes
Lunch: Barbecued Short Ribs
Dinner: Brussels Sprouts Casserole

Friday
Breakfast: Orange And Maple Syrup Quinoa
Lunch: Beer-braised Short Ribs
Dinner: Pasta And Mushrooms

Saturday
Breakfast: Vanilla And Nutmeg Oatmeal
Lunch: Lamb Stew
Dinner: Onion Cabbage

Sunday

Breakfast: Pecans Cake

Lunch: Barbecued Ham

Dinner: Cheese Broccoli

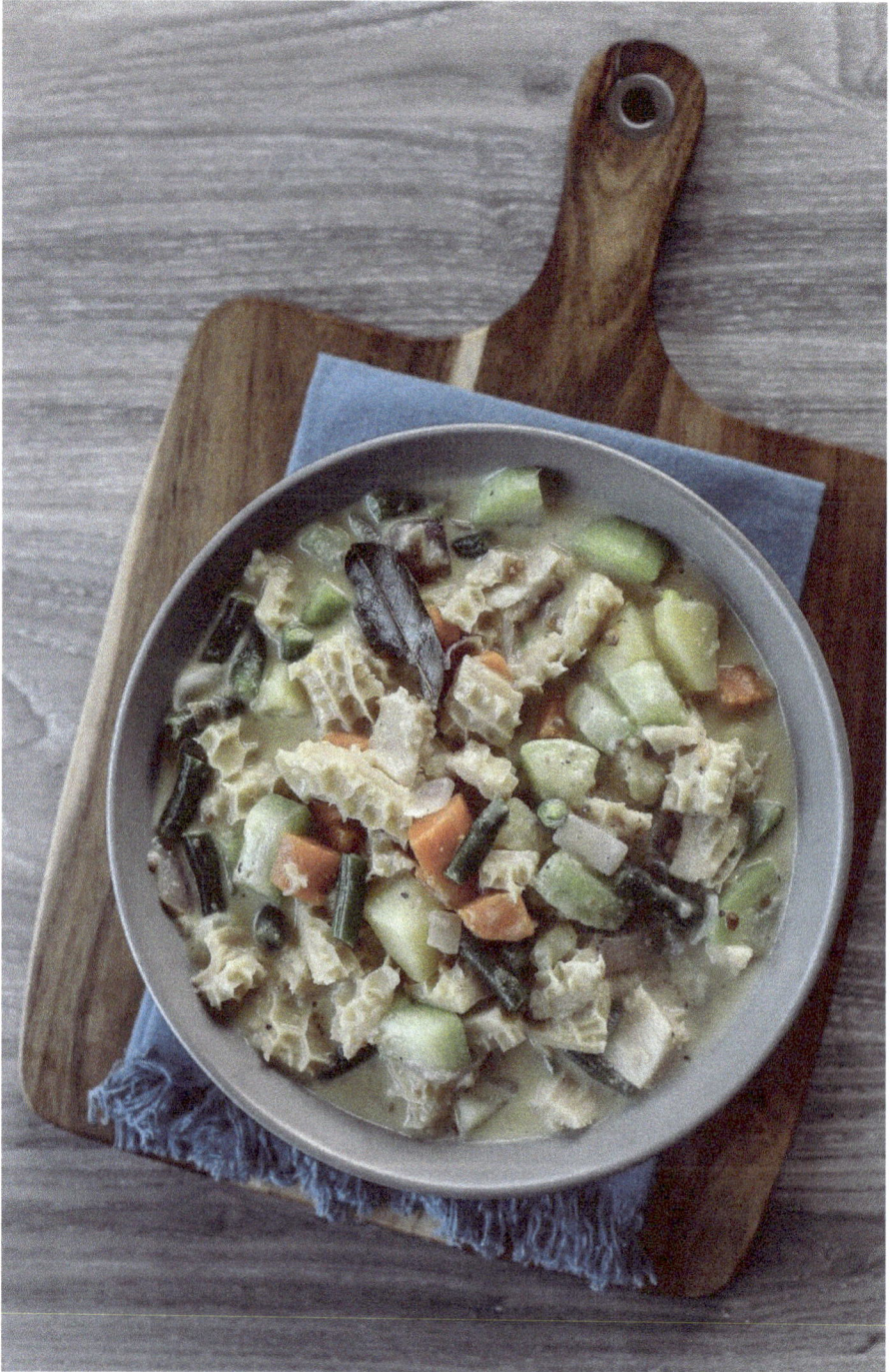